BODYWEIGHT TRAINING FOR WOMEN

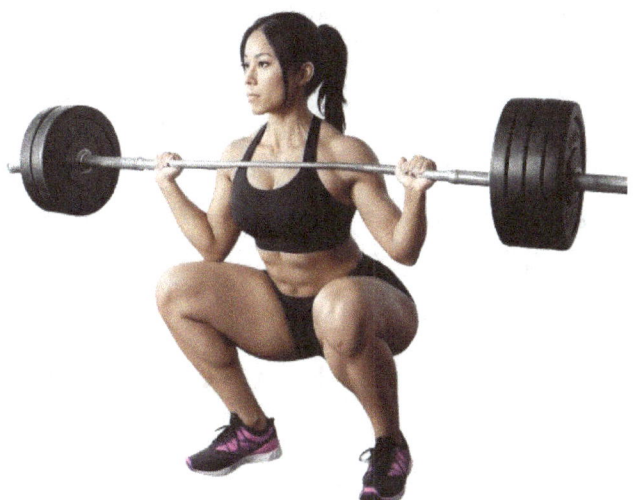

Proven At-Home Exercises for Building Strength and Losing Fat

RICHARD L. LYONS

This book is a work of nonfiction. The information and opinions expressed in this book are those of the author and do not necessarily reflect the views of the publisher.

!!!THANK YOU FOR PURCHASE THIS

GAIN ACCESS TO MORE BOOKS FROM ME

TABLE OF CONTENT

INTRODUCTION

Lisa had struggled with her weight her whole life. Though she was active in high school sports, when she went off to college the freshman fifteen hit her hard. By 25 she carried an extra 50 pounds on her 5'4" frame. She lacked energy, got winded going up stairs, and had constant back pain.

On a trip to the beach with friends, Lisa broke down seeing photos of herself looking unhealthy and overweight. She knew something had to change. When her friend Abby introduced her to bodyweight training, it gave her the tools she needed to reinvent herself.

Lisa started slowly - a 15 minute core routine while watching TV, a few sets of squats before showering. As she gained strength, Abby challenged her to longer bodyweight workouts 4 times a week. Lisa saw muscle definition in her arms and legs she never had before. The burning during plank holds got easier. After 3 months she could do full push ups and piston-like squat jumps.

In a year Lisa shed 20 pounds and kept it off. She still does her bodyweight circuits which give her energy, keep her back pain-free, and tone her into the best shape of her life. She feels stronger and healthier than she did even as a teen athlete.

Lisa says: "I wish I had discovered how empowering bodyweight training was years ago! I cannot express enough gratitude for how it has transformed my health, self-confidence and lifestyle."

GET LEAN AND STRONG WITH BODYWEIGHT TRAINING

If you cringe when you pass by the weights section of a gym, you're not alone. Lifting heavy barbells surrounded mostly by men can feel intimidating. The good news is that sculpting your dream physique doesn't require scary equipment or even a gym membership. Bodyweight workouts are extremely effective for building women's strength, burning fat, and revealing those toned abs every magazine cover seems to flaunt.

Basics of Bodyweight Training

Bodyweight training, also called bodyweight resistance training, utilizes your own body to provide resistance against gravity. Instead of relying on free weights, machines, or resistance bands, the resistance comes from your body working against itself in movements like planks, squats, lunges, pushups and more. The benefits are vast:

- Convenient - no gym or equipment needed, just basic space
- Efficient - works multiple muscle groups simultaneously
- Adaptable - easily modified for any fitness level
- Functional - mimics real life movements
- Economical - zero financial investment required
- Effective - builds lean muscle and burns calories comparable to weight lifting

Whether your goals are weight loss, overall fitness, or that bikini body, a bodyweight routine can get you there without an expensive gym membership or confusing strength training equipment. Let's explore why bodyweight training delivers such drastic body transformation results for women.

Building Lean Muscle

Most women avoid weight lifting from fear of getting "too bulky". Yet lifting weights is precisely what shapes a toned, feminine physique. The method works by progressively overloading and challenging the muscles so they adapt and get stronger. Added lean muscle boosts your metabolism, allowing you to burn more calories 24/7. Unlike cardio which only burns calories during a workout, extra muscle keeps your body burning fat while sitting at your desk, sleeping, walking - basically all day long!

Here is the incredible part - bodyweight training builds lean muscle just as efficiently as those intimidating barbells! Resisting your own body weight in multi-plane movements forces the same muscle adaptation. As you become stronger, you simply change leverage, angles, or add reps to keep challenging those muscles to grow. Core moves like pushups, squats, and lunges done with progressive overload sculpt lean definition.

Torching Fat

Cardio has another benefit too - it burns LOTS of calories and fat. Running, biking, and bootcamp classes get your heart rate sky-high. The more winded and sweaty you get, the more calories melt off your frame during and after your workout. But who has time and energy for an exhausting spin class daily??

The underappreciated secret is that bodyweight training provides an incredible calorie and fat burn too. The compound movements by nature require more muscle recruitment and effort. A few sets of mountain climbers, skaters, jumping jacks, or holding a plank already has you huffing and puffing. As your workout time with bodyweight exercises creeps towards the 30-60 minute range, your metabolism gets cranked for hours afterwards. This "afterburn effect" means fat continues melting off long after you towel off. For time-strapped women aiming for maximum fat loss with limited gym time, it is hard to beat bodyweight training's efficiency.

Confidence and Community

Beyond physical changes, bodyweight training boosts women's confidence and connectedness with their bodies. By mastering challenging moves like handstands, pullups, or advanced abs sequences, you gain self-assurance and pride. Bodyweight training lets you tap into steadfast perseverance. Hitting new rep records or advancing into more difficult progressions creates genuine self-esteem unrelated to unrealistic images on Instagram.

Plus a whole sisterhood exists cheering each other on! Facebook groups, Youtube channels, and women supporting women abound in the bodyweight space. It lacks the exclusivity of trendy boutique gyms or clique-ishness of Crossfit boxes. Just everyday women crushing fitness goals together creates positive ripple effects benefitting self-image and body positivity for all shapes and sizes.

Convinced of the merits? Keep reading to explore:

- Essential equipment to create your at-home gym
- Dynamic warmups to prevent injury
- Foundational movement patterns and progressions
- Creative cardio routines that annihilate fat
- Gentle cooldowns and self-care

You CAN have it all - strength, confidence, community and a rockin' physique with bodyweight training! Commit to the basics in this program, stick with it, and watch your transformation unfold!

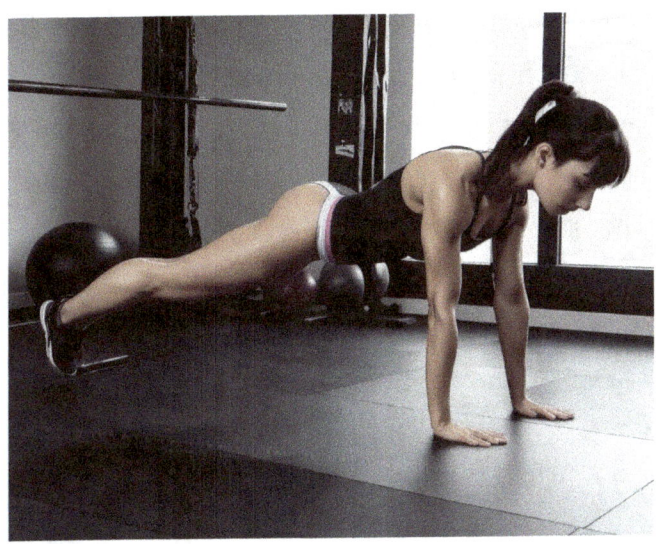

CHAPTER 1

CREATING YOUR HOME BODYWEIGHT GYM

Before diving into killer workout routines to sculpt lean muscle and torch calories, laying the foundation for training at home is key. Setting up your personal gym space thoughtfully will make bodyweight workouts efficient, safe, and enjoyable. This chapter covers:

- Evaluating room options
- Essential equipment
- Floor cushioning
- Using household items for resistance training

- Organization strategies

Let's tackle transforming your domestic domain into a fully-equipped training zone!

Choosing a Workout Area

Look around your home with fresh eyes for underutilized areas prime for conversion into workout spaces. Seek open floor plans without clutter to allow performing exercises safely. Here are elements to consider:

Living Rooms:

Offer generous dimensions but furniture obstacles exist. Ensure adequate clearance from coffee tables when performing stretching or movements like burpees. Mount TVs high enough to avoid collision during mountain climbers.

Bedrooms:

Another common default option, though often more compact. Position workout gear away from floor lamps or low windows to prevent kicking accidentally mid-jumping jacks. Just beware wincing family members above downstairs ceilings.

Basements / Finished Attics:
Offer blank canvases for constructing custom home gyms. Watch for sloped ceilings blocking overhead movements in attics. Basements with concrete floors enable seamless mounting of equipment but evaluate mustiness or temperature extremes.

Garages:
Provide ample square footage but possibly lack climate control. Ensure exhaust fans ventilate fumes during high intensity sessions. Position gear away from tool benches to avoid loose hardware underfoot.

Outdoor Spaces:
Bring the indoors outside when weather permits. Decks, patios or yards extend options but contend with temperature swings and precipitation. Avoid slippery surfaces and inground sprinkler heads.

Once your training zone is established, optimize further by:

- Adding mirrors to check form
- Mounting wall hooks for resistance bands
- Incorporating scenic views for motivation
- Playing energizing music
- Creating splash zones safe from sweat droplets

Essential Bodyweight Gear

Owning extensive equipment is totally unnecessary. However investing in a few key items makes training more comfortable, efficient and injury-proof.

Yoga Mats:

These grippy thin pads cushion against hard floors for floor exercises. Look for antimicrobial versions if sharing space. I love Manduka Pros or Lululemon reversible mats.

Foam Roller:

Rolling out tight muscles pre or post workout aids recovery and reduces soreness. Textured styles provide trigger point release too. Major winners are Rumblerollers and Hyperice Vyper models.

Resistance Bands:

These stretchy elastic bands in varying resistance levels add challenge to movements. Loop bands around wrists/ankles during routines or safely anchor bands for pull exercises. Top brands are Rogue, Fit Simplify, and Whatafit.

Ab Wheel:

Wicked core strengthener that rolls out from knees, intensifying planks. Choose models with knee pads like the Perfect Fitness Ab Carver Pro or Athlean-X Ab wheel.

Jump Rope:

My favorite cardio calorie-burner engages shoulders, arms and calves simultaneously. Weighted or adjustable ropes allow customization for harder hiit-style training. I recommend Crossrope, Rx Smart Gear or Sonic Boom M2 ropes.

Timer:

Crucial for tracking rest intervals, setting timed circuits or tabata sequences. Digital timers like Timex or Gymboss allow preprogramming multi-interval workouts. Most smartphone fitness apps sync with watches too.

Heart Rate Monitor:

Telemetric chest straps like Polar H10 provide constant pulse tracking during intense metcon or HIIT training. Sync with equipment like Concept 2 rower for fat burn accuracy.

The above basic bodyweight gear costs under $300 total and lasts for years. Now let's explore economical alternatives using common household items.

Household Resistance Tools

Part of body weight training's appeal lies in not requiring paid gym memberships or expensive equipment purchases.Odds are you own numerous ready-to-grab items which add resistance during workouts. Explore your pantry, garage and basement for handy tools like:

Canned Goods: Bicep curls, lateral raises, front raises. Heavier weights work core and legs too.

- Milk Jugs: Fill with sand/water/rocks for curls, rows, overhead presses. Duct tape securely closed after filling.
- Backpacks: Load with books for weighted pushups, step ups, lunges or squats. Adjust weight as possible.
- Towels: Drape over pull up bars for easier gripping doing pull ups or inverted rows.
- Brooms/Mops: Hold horizontally and perform trap raises, bicep curls, tricep extensions. Vary grips for balance challenges too.
- Resistance bands: Loop bands around furniture legs for attaching slide bands, assisting pull up progression, or increasing squat difficulty.
- Chairs: Incline pushups, triceps dips, step ups. Also useful for band anchor points.

- Countertops: Triceps dips using kitchen or bathroom cabinets. Be sure surfaces are secured properly first.
- Couch Cushions: Place under chest or feet during incline/decline pushups. Also handy for elevating feet during crunches or leg lifts.

Balancing on cushions while performing squats engages stabilizer muscles more also.

As your strength increases, swap household tools for heavier weights or more challenging resistance band tensions. This saves money until investing in more specialized equipment makes sense.

Now let's optimize organization.

Get Organized

Finally, staying organized maximizes your home gym experience while minimizing clutter. Simple strategies like:
- Labelling storage bins for gear types
- Hanging foam rollers/resistance bands on wall hooks

- Coiling jump ropes on mounted dowels
- Displaying motivational quotes/photos
- Assigning specific zones for strength, cardio, etc
- Using woven baskets for towel storage
- Investing in an anti-fatigue workout mat

Transforms wasted spaces into welcoming workout havens. Our homes contain hidden gems perfect for outfitting our own bodyweight studios. A bit of trial and error to customize your zone alongside foundational equipment gets your environment fully prepped for sweat sessions ahead. Time to put your refined training habitat to work transforming your body one rep at a time!

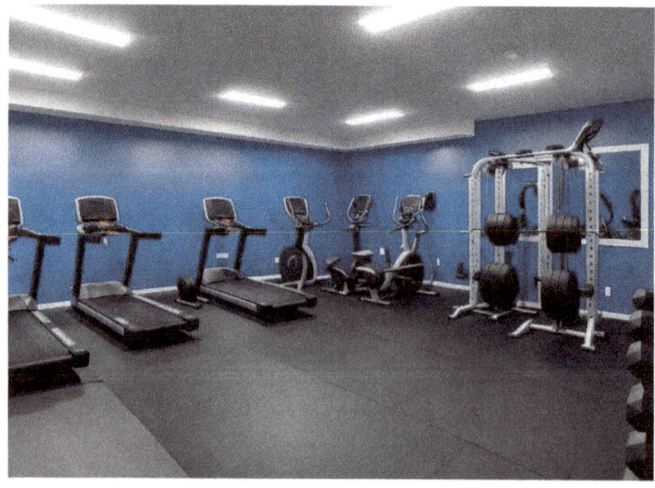

CHAPTER 2

LIMBERING UP - ESSENTIAL WARMUPS AND STRETCHING

Before plunging into hardcore strength circuits or high intensity cardio, properly warming up prepares muscles, increases joint range of motion, and prevents injury. Think of warmups as the onramp accelerating workout performance and keeping bodies resilient long-term. We dive into:

- Warmup benefits
- Dynamic movements
- Static stretching
- Yoga-inspired flows
- Sport-specific routines

Let's explore essential prep work enabling you to train vigorously while dodging doctor's office visits!

Why Bother Warming Up?

Warming up readies the body for exercise by literally raising muscle temperature and blood flow. Think of your muscles as elastic bands - gold bands snap when stretched versus warm bands with pliability to move freely through a full range of motion.

Specifically, properly warming up:

- Increases range of motion
- Heightens nerve impulse conduction
- Elevates oxygen delivery to muscles
- Reduces risk of strains or tears
- Enhances motor neuron excitability
- Improves power and strength output
- Ups endurance and stamina

We all learned those middle school calisthenics before blitzing the track or court. But modern protocols moved beyond lackadaisical arm circles or haphazard toe touches. Today's progressive exercises prepare players for the rapid start-stop motions and cutting common in their sports.

Let's demonstrate working up an elevated heart rate using full body movements.

Dynamic Warm Ups

Dynamic stretches utilize constant motion through progressive ranges unlike static stretching holding singular sustained poses. Think high knees, inchworms and other repetitive drills raising core body temperature.

The goal is teaching proper movement patterns while increasing demands on the muscles with flowing sequences. Begin general then evolve warm up towards specific activities ahead.

General Full Body Activation

First raise your heart rate for 2-3 minutes performing light calisthenics like:

- Jogging with arm swings

- Jumping jacks
- Skip knees high
- Shoot basketball layups (no ball needed)
- Punch outs with high steps

Then begin sequencing multiple planes of motion with challenges like:

- High knee grabs
- Frankensteins
- Heel kicks
- Bear crawls
- Lateral shuffles
- Cariocas

Progress by adding tempo changes - fast feet then holding a squat before the next move. Conclude this general warmup stretching major muscle groups.

Sport Specific Warmups
Cater warmups towards upcoming activities whether battering up softball swings or rehearsing dance choreography at 50% tempo.

Some examples:

- Golfers: Rotate through torso, mobilize shoulders exaggerating backswings.

- Yogis: Sun salutations slowly then holding Downward Dog, melting into hips and hamstrings.

- Runners: Walk lunges, inchworms, leg swings, gradual accelerating strides.

- CrossFit: Light deadlifts, air squats, presses, mobilizing major joints through range of motion.

- Dancers: Iterate through routine at half pace, pulse stretches in splits, pikes and straddles.

- Weight Trainers: Bodyweight or banded squats, pulling resistance bands, intermediate planks focusing on form.

Adapt this sport specificity to any upcoming endeavors but don't overlook static stretching too.

Static Stretching

While dynamic moves raise body temp, holding extended static stretches increases flexibility and joint mobility. After general warmups, spend another 5-10 minutes working into deeper classic stretches.

Focus on major muscle groups like:
- Calves - Downward Dog variations
- Hamstrings - Seated or standing forward folds
- Hips / Glutes - Figure 4, Frog pose, Pigeon pose
- Quadriceps / Hip Flexors - Standing or kneeling lunge variations
- Chest / Shoulders - Child's pose
- Upper back - Cat / Camel poses
- Lats - Standing side bends

Progress intensity stretching each muscle 2-3 times on each side. Breathe steadily into tight areas without compromising form. Use props like yoga blocks to release deeper into holds.

After working major muscle groups, conclude with full body sequences borrowing from yoga flows.

Yoga Warmup Flows

Link individual static stretches into smooth sequences - great for dancers, barre or pilates practitioners. Flows increase mobility, alignment and mind-body connection.

Some starter yoga flows may include:
- Child's pose into Downward Facing Dog into Standing Forward Fold sequence x 5 breaths each
- Triangle pose flowing to Half-Moon pose to Warrior 2 sequence x 5 breaths each side
- Seated spinal twists both directions into gentle backbends like Camel pose or Bridge pose

Check your ego during dedicated warm up periods. The priority lies properly preparing structures for work ahead - not showing off. Warmups lay the critical foundation for stellar training sessions. Show your body TLC ensuring every workout begins to set up for victory.

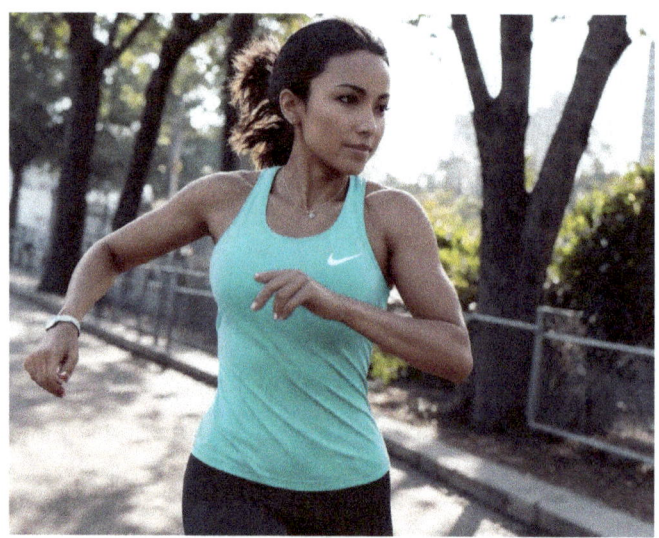

CHAPTER 3

CORE STRENGTH - SCULPTING A POWERFUL MIDSECTION

Defined abdominal muscles represent more than vanity. A strong inner core stabilizes your entire body for greater efficiency, power transfer and injury resilience when playing sports or performing routine activities alike. Core training sculpts a trim waistline plus aids better posture and spinal alignment.

We explore popular staples plus creative challenges for obliques, lower abs, and that coveted six pack:

- Core essentials

- Plank progressions
- Advanced crunches
- Oblique shredders
- Underused lifts
- Putting it all together

Time to carve your dream midsection from all angles!

Core Training Basics

Your core encompasses over 30 muscles spanning from hips to shoulders stabilizing the spine, pelvis and torso. Major players include:

- Rectus abdominis - Vertical 6 pack muscles
- Obliques - Rotational muscles along each side
- Transverse abdominis - Innermost corset muscle
- Erector spinae - Flanking upper back muscles

Classic crunches or situps target the 6 pack's rectus abdominis effectively. However, directly working the deeper transverse abdominis better supports the low back and alignment. Forget gadgets - bodyweight at the proper progressions trains core endurance safely.

Plank Progressions

Perhaps nothing reveals core fitness (or weakness!) more than the basic plank hold. Simply holding your body stiff as a board belly down engages those stabilizers isometrically. Most Physical therapists consider planks the gold standard since the position trains endurance in neutral spinal alignment safely.

Since planks remain static, their simplicity invites creativity in progressions:

- Increase intensity by elevating feet onto chair seats. Higher difficulty!

- Walk feet wider than closer together to fire inner thighs too.

- Lift one arm or leg in "chorus line" kicks. Teases stabilizers!

- Add diagonal arm/leg lifts staying rigid in the center. Much harder than just holding!

- Place a pillow under elbows for incline planks. Ouch.

- Rotate planks sideways into walls initially. Gradually increase time.

- Once strong, test Renegade planks with rotator cuff work holding light dumbbells.

Planks strengthen the entire body in proper alignment - yet only require a mat showing their versatility. Keep perfect form, take breaks to maintain a rigid spine, and incrementally build hold times towards 3-5 minutes.

For cheap abs definition also include weighted crunches and leg raises.

Killer Crunches

Who doesn't aspire for that elusive 6 pack? While planks fortify the core, adding isolation exercises tones each ab "block". Decline weights during crunches or cable crunches hammer those rectus muscles efficiently. Some crunching variations include:

- Bicycle crunches with alternating elbow to opposite knee
- Cross body jackknife crunches touching elbow beyond center
- Twisted rope crunches holding a medicine ball
- Feet elevated crunches hoisting legs up at angle

Intensity options:
- Increase reps for muscular endurance
- Explode during concentric, control eccentrics
- Add weight plates or dumbbells across chest
- Attach bands above head for constant tension

- Use ab wheel for max range of motion

Crunches develop coveted 6 pack definitions. Now work the lower abs and obliques with leg lifts and rotational moves.

Oblique Obliterators

The obliques span from love handles up behind the ribcage controlling side to side spinal motions. Chisel the obliques adding slow and controlled rotational work like:

- Russian twists: Keeping abs braced, rotate holding plate, slam ball or medball
- Seated trunk rotations: Anchor stretch band to stable object, rotate away working against resistance
- Standing cable chops: Pull high to low diagonally across body
- Landmine 180 rotations: Squat rotating under suspended barbell

Use control emphasizing the contraction and resisting momentum. Lighter weights with mind-muscle connection beats heaving and momentum.

Now lift your legs, not just weights!

Leg Lifts and Extensions

Lower ab exercises lift legs up working against gravity rather than pulling the torso down crunching. Leg raises like:

- Hanging leg lifts: Grip pull up bar raising straight legs
- Decline bench leg raises: Brace back on incline, raise/lower legs
- Flutter kicks: Hold legs off floor alternating up/down small pulses

Also horizontal moves like:
- Dragon flags: Supporting torso on bench, lift legs keeping them straight
- Reverse crunches: Raise knees to chest while lying back
- Banded good mornings: Anchor band around back, hinge forward

Emphasize control, incremental raises, and steady eccentric lowering without slamming feet to floor. Those often neglected lower abdominals contribute hugely toward reversing that abdominal pooch!

Programming it All Together

Choose 2-4 core moves through the various categories above. Sequence together into circuits or mini-supersets for time then rest intervals. This stimulates core endurance while allowing muscles to recover before subsequent sets.

Sample Core Workouts:

5 Rounds:

1) 30 second plank hold into 10 crunches

Rest 30 seconds between rounds

3 Supersets:

A) 15 Reverse crunches / 15 bicycle crunches

B) 30 second side planks left / 30 second side planks right

Rest 30-45 seconds between paired sets

Straight Sets:

12 Russian Twists with 8 kg slam ball

15 Cable lifts with 5kg plate

10 Decline bench leg raises

Rest 60 seconds between straight sets

That rock solid core and finally visible abs await your dedication. Mix and match elements working center stabilizers then isolated muscles for ultimate core development. Say bye to that belly pooch and hello to enviable core definition!

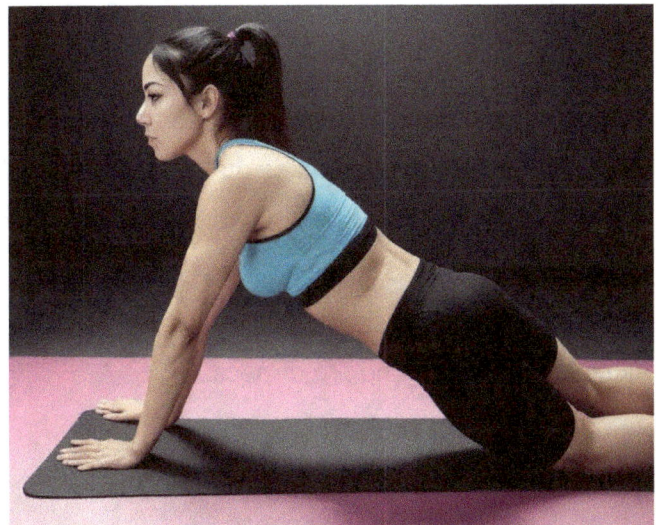

CHAPTER 4

PUSHING TO POWER - CONQUERING PUSH-UPS AND CHEST STRENGTH

Reclaiming the ability to perform full pushups proves empowering. Standard floor pushups utilize 64% of total body muscle mass making them one of the most efficient functional exercises. Continually progressing by adding repetitions or introducing variations transforms flabby arms into toned triceps, sculpted shoulders and firmer pecs.

This chapter explores:
- Benefits beyond the chest
- Push up progressions
- Advanced variations

- Equipment elevations
- Dips and supplemental work

Let's tackle mastering push up dominance!

Pushing Past Weakness

If struggling through a single toe-touching, back-dipping push up sounds familiar, you're not alone. With desk jobs and device scrolling the norm, our upper body pushing strength often declines prematurely. However incremental progressions using inclined angles, wall pushups and knee variations lead to eventual floor push up success.

Strengthening the upper body provides practical strength for daily tasks like lifting kids or groceries more easily. Who doesn't want that?

Globally, pushups open the doorway as the perfect beginner compound exercise. Once initiated, adding reps after each workout constructs upper body capability literally from the ground up. Using sturdy boxes, benches, chairs or even bathroom countertops as platforms allows gradually working towards the floor. Beginning elevated trains proper shoulder, core and leg stabilization making the eventual transition off supports more seamless.

Set a goal like 10-20 quality pushups straight without compromising form. Be patient in scaled progressions but persistent in regular attempts multiple times weekly. Let's walk through common variations:

Incline Push Ups
The most beginner-friendly push up version starts feet on floor with hands elevated on a box, bench, or step. This reduces resistance to about 70% of a standard push up's demands. As strength increases, eventually graduate box height decreases towards the ground.

Wall Push Ups
Facing any flat vertical surface like a wall allows another inclined option. Stand in front, lean forward placing palms shoulder width on the wall and

perform the push up motion. Start with high reps here before progressing.

Knee Push Ups

From all fours, leave knees grounded as you perform the push up normally. Reducing the lever length lightens resistance to make repetitions possible. Over time, begin straightening one leg slowly at a time until both extend during full plank push ups.

Negatives / Partial ROM

Can perform a few push ups but lack the strength completing higher reps? Introduce "negatives" - resisting while lowering only.

From the plank, take 3 seconds lowering until the chest touches the floor. Hold briefly before straight arm planking back upward. Or try increasing reps by limiting range of motion - perform the mid-portion only without fully locking or touching the ground.

Advanced Floor Variations

Once mastering straight repetitions, additional challenges await:

- Staggered hands: Widen or alternate one hand forward/back to increase chest tension

- Diamond push ups: Narrow hands together under chest emphasizing triceps

- Fingertip push ups: Balance weight through hands without full palm contact

- Dive bomber push ups: Begin in Downward Dog, swoop chest forward between arms to Chaturanga plank before upward press

- One arm push ups: Hoist other hand in the air for crazy strength and stabilization!

Equipment elevations

Add dumbbells under each palm or place each hand atop 2-3 aerobics steps. Suspension trainers like TRX bands also angle hands lower than toes forcing increased effort. Dips leverage gymnastics rings or benches too for concentrated triceps burn!

The journey to push up mastery challenges adults physically and mentally alike. But nothing substitutes finally achieving well-earned, hard fought strength gains. And that toned upper body becomes a badge of tenacity! Keep pressing play by adding variety when strength plateaus. Push up dominance awaits!

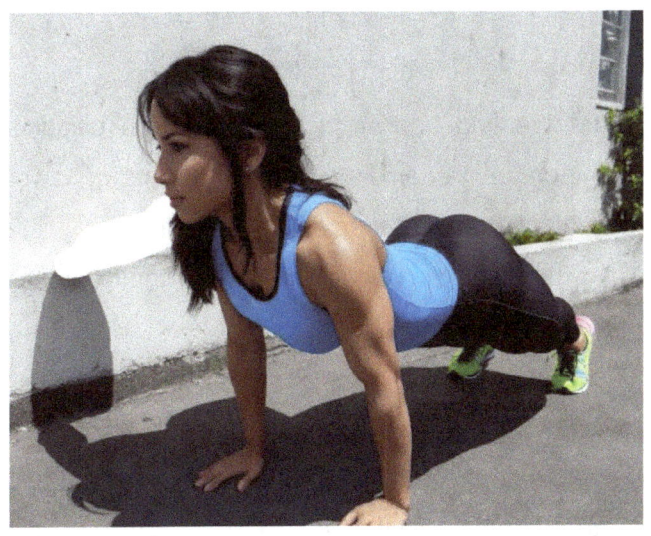

CHAPTER 5

LOWER BODY SCULPTORS - SQUATS, LUNGES AND LEG BLISS

Forget wasting hours slogging away on elliptical machines or treadmills. Want to transform lower body weakness into enviable athletic legs fast? Make friends with squats, lunges and their endless challenging variants!

Lower body training not only reduces thigh or glute flab, it floods muscles with growth promoting hormones while skyrocketing calorie burn too. Lift heavier with the largest muscle groups for maximum body recomposition effects. We explore foundational movements plus creative blends targeting quads, hamstrings, glutes and calves:

- Mastering Squats
- Lunges 101
- Single Leg Exercises
- Glute Activators
- Calf Specialization
- Advanced Aerobic Leg Burners

Grab the oversized hoodie to disguise quad and hammy soreness sure to follow - we're taking legs to school!

PERFECTING SQUATS

Mastering proper squat form marks a pivotal milestone before introducing more exotic or loaded variations. Initiate each rep by unlocking the hips back, allowing knees to track over toes while keeping weight predominantly in the heels. Descend until thighs reach parallel with kneecaps aligned over feet. Many squat struggles originate from immobilized ankles or hips - remain weighty through each heel keeping knees pressing outward not inward.

While balancing mobility, ensure proper spinal alignment by:

- Keeping core braced
- Chin tilted slightly upwards
- Elbows wide aiming to raise hands overhead (even if mobility restricts)
- Knees always tracking in same direction as toes
- Avoiding butt wink or excessive forward leaning

Once comfortable through 20-30 bodyweight reps, progress load or complexity.

Adding Resistance
Wrap mini-resistance bands just above knees or hold dumbbells at shoulder height when mobility allows. Execute slow and controlled for increased time under tension. Over time add plates across the

upper back or shoulders once confident balancing heavier loads.

Vary Foot Positions

Turn toes out into a sumo squat firing inner thighs more. Stagger one foot forward into a Bulgarian split squat isolating each leg individually. Elevate heels onto 10-15 lb plates improving ankle dorsiflexion.

Explode Upward

Introduce jump squats leaving the ground explosively to integrate power. Land softly back into the squat pocket to reinforce positional strength and save joints.

Now lunge ahead into ultimate leg immolation!

Lunge Litmus Test

Lunges function as both stability drills and quad destroyers. Step one leg forward, descending until the rear knee nearly kisses the floor. Ensure the front knee remains centered over the ankle, never drifting inward. Proper hip hinge determines depth able to replicate without torso compromise.

When comfortable through basic lunge patterns, unleash creative variants like:

- Bulgarian Split Squat (rear elevated on bench)
- Walking Lunges holding weights
- Reverse Lunges stepping backward
- Lateral Lunges to each side
- Curtsy Lunges crossing behind lead leg
- Jumping Lunges launching airborne

The stretch reflex engaging the anterior quad before simultaneously recruiting the posterior glute makes lunges ridiculously effective when executed properly. Use only bodyweight initially before loading progression since technique remains paramount.

Now drop down isolating just one leg at a time.

Single Leg Exercises

Unilateral moves magnify leg deficits since the non-working leg cannot compensate for weaknesses. Challenge coordination going single leg with moves like:

- Pistol Squats
- Shrimp Squats
- Single Leg Deadlifts
- Skater Hops
- Step Ups onto box

Balancing while resisting body weight or weights improves stability and strength too. Avoid turning these into momentum-based plyometric drills before mastering controlled constant tension execution first. Master the basics before chasing flashy hybrids on Instagram.

Now loop around activating backside glutes and hams.

Glute Glory
The maximus constitutes the largest muscle in the body. Want depth, roundness and lift to your rump?

Train endurance first before chasing crazy resistance levels. Glute bridges transition well from planks:

- Hip Thrusters (shoulder elevated version)
- Donkey Kicks
- Glute Bridges
- Fire Hydrants
- Clamshells with resistance bands

Emphasize the top squeeze contracting glutes fully. Increase difficulty elevating opposite arm/leg or feet during extensions. Feeling extra spicy? Grab the barbell for weighted variations after perfecting form through high reps.

Calf Complements
Finally carve diamond shaped calves with dedicated isolation work. Perform standing calf raises:

- Single leg
- Unilateral difference stances like sumo
- Explosive rebounds off a box

- Seated calf raises using leg press machine

Vary foot positions and contraction methods - flexed toes, externally rotated - to spur ongoing adaptation. Now let's fuse strength with sweaty conditioning completing our leg day lesson!

Metabolic Leg Burners

Combine lower body resistance with intense cardio spikes for maximum fat scorching while driving muscular endurance sky high. Think squat thrust burpees, lateral shuffle jumps over cones, and reverse lunges down full basketball courts. Introduce equipment as tolerable for added difficulty:

- Jumping box drills
- Lateral hurdle hops
- Agility ladder shuffle runs
- Mountain climber switch kicks
- Jump rope drills between weighted Goblet squats

Completing 2-4 sets of 30-60 seconds all-out effort makes sprawling on the mat involuntarily tempting. But our diligence cultivating full leg development bears delicious fruit in the form of athletic leanness, mobility and amplified athleticism...not to mention that complementary curvaceous backside too!

Dare to squat below parallel, split stance with pride and bare those massively developed legs as badges of honor from months of progressive overload. Now who's ready to attack leg day? Let's get it!!

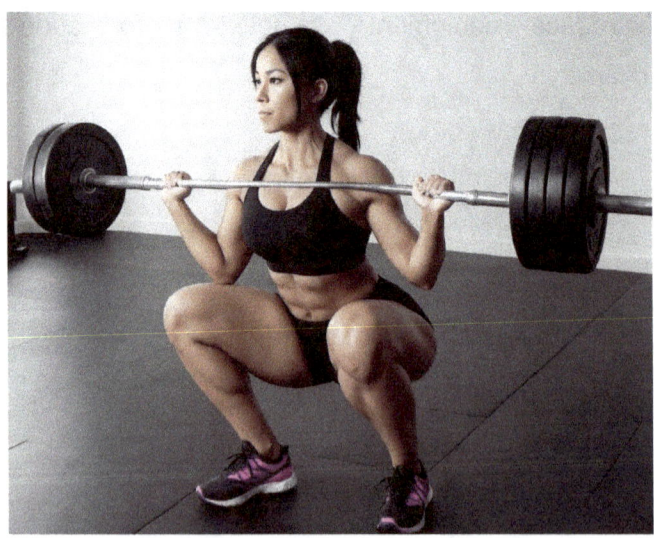

CHAPTER 6

BUILD YOUR BEST BUTT - SCULPTED GLUTES AND HIP WORKOUTS

Let's be real. Who doesn't aspire to upgrade their backside with more lift, roundness and tone? Call it athleticism or sexuality, sculpted glutes undeniably transform physiques and boost confidence. Fortunately the largest muscle group in the body responds incredibly well to targeted training. So let's craft coveted curves you can't help but show off!

This booty makeover chapter will:
- Explain glute anatomy
- Prioritize activation

- Progress hip thrusts
- Introduce uncommon isolators
- Spice things up with variety

Let's analyze how to best build, lift and amplify your ultimate asset!

Glute Anatomy Basics

The gluteal region constitutes three distinct muscles:

- Gluteus Maximus – Big daddy muscle spanning from low back to upper thigh responsible for hip extension and external rotation. Makes up the bulk and roundness of the backside shape.

- Gluteus Medius – Located underneath max along pelvis and thigh bone maintaining hip stability and abduction away from midline when walking or rotating. Prevents knees collapsing inward.

- Gluteus Minimus – Furthest undersurface glute being smaller than medius. Works synchronously controlling subtle hip and pelvis motions.

This trio of stacked muscles interworking together form the envy of backsides everywhere when properly trained for roundness, stability and strength through full ranges. Let's wake them up first before sculpting the shape.

Activating Glutes

Many glute workouts excessively target the bigger gluteus maximus using bridge variations while neglecting the smaller stability-focused medius and minimus muscles. This imbalance often manifests as excessive knee valgus (inward knee collapse), hip shifts in planks or squats, and low back discomfort from improper pelvic positioning.

Try this quick test: lay on your back with one knee bent, other leg extended. Can you lift your straightened leg a few inches without the bent knee dropping out or inward? Be honest! This screens for baseline glute medius and minimus function responsible for stabilizing the femur properly.

If your leg remains aligned, congratulations! For most women however, hip rotator and core weakness manifest until addressed. Let's build proper hip function with targeted mini-band side walks targeting smaller glute medius/minimus muscles first before leaping into hyper glute max training.

Basic hip activation exercises include
- Mini-band monster walks
- Lateral leg raises
- Clam shells
- Donkey kicks
- Ice skaters

Focus on quality reps with full range of motion and honest self-assessment. Can't properly activate glutes initially? Perfect - identifying limitations helps guide needs specific programming. Now let's start building shape with hip thrusts!

Level Up Hip Thrusters

Barbell hip thrusts explosively strengthen glutes with the added perk of zero spinal loading making them lower back friendly. Here is solid progression model:

Phase 1 - Bodyweight

Focus first on mind-muscle connection using only body weight for 1-2 weeks. Squeeze glutes forcefully pausing each rep at the top position.

Phase 2 - Band Resistance

Loop thicker bands above knees or anchor longer bands around the bar/pillar for extra pull. Use lighter tensions focusing again on top range peak contraction.

Phase 3 - Weight Plate Addition

Balance starting around a 25 lb plate on hips for beginner women building adequate strength to control heavier loads. Avoid going overly heavy initially - intensity via volume proves most efficient here.

Phase 4 - Barbell Progression

Now holding an unweighted Olympic barbell or EZ Curl bar across hips, begin adding smaller 1-2 lb plates weekly aiming for 3-4 sets of 8-15 reps adding monthly weight conservatively.

This patient model allows connective tissues adapting to progressive overload avoiding risky sharp spikes in intensity. Now complement hip thrusters with isolation exercises.

Targeted Isolation Moves

Balancing horizontal hip extension patterns, include additional planes of movement hitting each glute muscle uniquely:

Vertical - Squats, stepped lunges

Lateral - Side lying clam shells, banded walks, monster walks, side steps

Rotational - Seated band abduction, cable kickbacks or chop rotations

Sample follow-along Supersets:

A1) Barbell Hip Thruster - 4 sets x 6-10 reps

A2) Walking Side Lunges - 4 sets x 8-12 reps each leg

B1) Sliding Lateral Leg Raises - 3 sets x 12-15 reps each leg

B2) Quadruped Fire Hydrants - 3 sets x 15-20 reps each leg

These contrasting movements better stimulate overall glute growth compared to repetitive singular exercises alone. Change programming every 4-6 weeks to spur ongoing size and strength gains.

Now for some sassy workout finishers!

Advanced Moves

Once mastering above progressions, earn bonus points mixing in advanced exercises. Carefully experiment with:

- Single leg hip thrusts
- Weighted donkey kicks
- Frog pumps with bands

- Cable rope kickbacks
- Wall supported glute bridges

Play with foot positions too - externally rotating hips or wider than hip width engage glute medius and minors differently.

Prioritizing patient progressive overload forges enviable backside development over time. But also showcase booty victories periodically with well-earned fitted dresses and heels. Your dedication to sculpting spectacular glutes deserves flaunting! Just don't be surprised by the extra attention your new asset suddenly attracts…

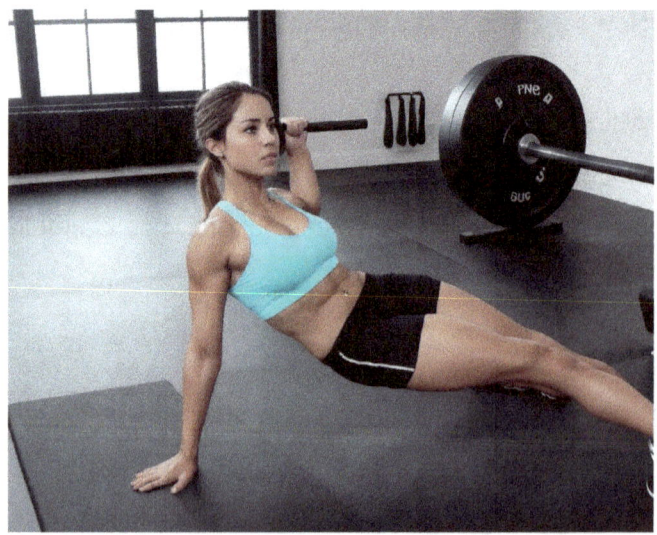

CHAPTER 7

SCULPTING STUNNING SHOULDERS AND ARMS

While lower body sweat sessions spike heart rates torching fat, let's not neglect upper bodies too. Well defined shoulders and toned arms not only boost appearance but translate to real world strength for functional movement, lifting groceries or hoisting small children!

Strategy remains key to building lean mass and avoiding bulky, masculine appearance women often dread. Follow below guidelines showcasing feminine physique enhancements, not overly ripped bodybuilder bodies requiring syringes. We explore:

- Shoulder anatomy
- Foundation exercises
- Arm isolations
- Rear shoulder carving
- Advanced push/pull supersets

Let's craft chiseled shoulders and defined arms befitting gorgeous goddesses!

Shoulder Girdle Basics

The shoulder spans four joints moving the arm utilizing muscles spanning the:

Front Deltoids: Lateral raises, front raises
Middle Deltoids: Presses, push ups, pike push ups
Rear Deltoids: Reverse flies, face pulls
Rotator Cuff: External/internal rotations

Balancing pushing and pulling volume keeps structures healthy. Avoiding behind the neck presses protects joints too. Warmups with bands or lightweight circles mobilize shoulders before heavier training. Let's build that iconic shoulder cap starting with push up progressions.

Push Up Foundations

Conquering push ups transforms flabby arms into toned triceps, firmer pecs and rounded deltoids popping. But avoid compromising alignment plunging straight to the floor using sloppy form. Try these on-ramp variations first:

- Wall push ups
- Incline push ups
- Kneeling push ups
- Eccentric lowering push ups

Once completing quality floor push ups, add intensity options like hand position changes:

- Wide grip
- Narrow / diamond
- Decline feet elevated
- Single arm (minor side assist)
- Fingertip push ups

Now complement horizontal pushing with vertical shoulder developers.

Shoulder Sculptors

Standing shoulder presses and lateral raises target deltoids with precision:

Overhead Presses: Dumbbell, barbell or single arm cable versions

Arnold Presses: Begin palms neutral pressing up then rotating externally lowering under control

Lateral Raises: Front, side, rear plane raises with perfect form - no momentum!

Now fire supports smaller stabilizer muscles with multi-plane motions.

Advanced Rotator Cuff Roasters

Balancing dominant muscle groups with external rotation exercises creates more balanced physiology and fewer overuse injuries:

Face pulls using suspension trainers or cables

Wall slides lowering controlled under tension then driving back upward

Band pull with elbows pulling wide against resistance

Bottoms-up kettlebell holds challenging grip stabilizers isometrically

With shoulders fire, let's shift downward to coveted defined arms next.

Arms Anatomy
The upper arm contains opposing muscles that straighten (triceps) and bend (biceps) the elbow joint while forearms rotate the wrists. Target all angles for complete development:

- Biceps - Arm curls
- Triceps - Underhand pushdowns
- Brachioradialis - Hammer curls

Forearms - Wrist curls, squeezes, carries

Now test true muscular endurance with high repetition burnouts!

Rep It Out Isolations

Nothing spikes metabolic stress and delivers swollen pumps like high repetition arm training. Use moderate weight totals allowing at least 15-20 reps to focus on muscle quality and increased capillary vascularization. Some ideas:

- Single arm preacher 21's (7 lower, 7 mid, 7 upper)
- Triple drop sets starting heavy then reducing weight

- Giant sets pairing biceps then immediately triceps without rest

- Ascending pyramids adding reps each successive set

Destroying individual arms with concentrated time under tension produces a coveted definition. But also integrate antagonists by supersetting opposing muscle groups.

Agonist Antagonist Supersets
Pre-fatigue before heavier compound moves with active contrast sequences like:

- Tricep pushdown drop sets into overhead dumbbell press

- Bicep spider curls preceding weighted pull ups

- Overhead tricep extensions before bench pressing

Pre-exhaustion engorges target muscles with blood saturation for rapid size gains when trained frequently. Vary grip widths, angles and equipment regularly to spur ongoing adaptations.

In summary sculpt defined arms and shoulders progressively in four strategic stages:

1) Perfect form through multiple planes targeting each head
2) Increase intensity once able (reps, load, tempo)
3) Isolate with high repetition blood volume techniques
4) Integrate agonist/antagonist supersets

Implementing above best practices avoids dangerous overuse injuries enabling healthy, alluring arm and shoulder punctuation. Who's ready to toss the cover up and proudly flaunt those earned physique upgrades? Let's get after it!

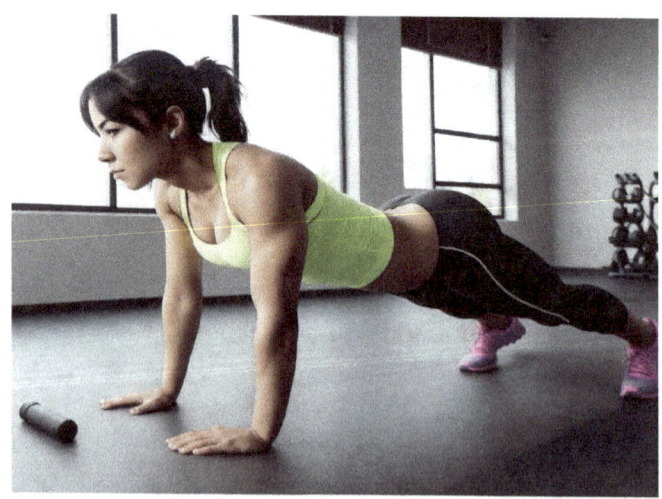

CHAPTER 8

EXPLOSIVE PLYOS - TORCHING FAT WITH JUMPS AND HOPS

When picturing quintessential fit physiques, lean and athletic comes to mind. Combining resistance training with targeted cardio blasts optimizes body composition. Why choose when certain exercises fuse strength AND sweat? Say hello to plyometrics!

This intense chapter adds:

- What defines plyometric training
- Safety first progressions
- Foundational movements
- Advanced variations

- Equipment elevations

Unleash your inner cardio bunny with heart pounding hops transforming bodies into ultimate calorie incinerating machines!

Plyometric Principles

Unlike traditional cardio sustaining heart rate with plodding miles, plyos spike power production taxing fuel sources quickly. The term plyometric implies strengthening muscles to unleash maximum force – in this case powerfully propelling your bodyweight explosively skyward!

Think bounding box jumps, skater hops, tuck jumps or vertical leaping. Each takeoff rapidly stretches muscle fibers followed by immediate tightening (stretch-shortening cycle) translating speed into airborne height or horizontal distance improvements.

Benefits include:
- Increased vertical leaping ability for sports
- Strengthen connective tissue resilience

- Improve neuromuscular coordination and balance
- Shoot metabolism sky-high burning tons of calories

When programmed strategically alongside resistance training, plyos transform bodies into ultimate fat shredding machines!

Safety First

As with any ballistic activity, technique trump's testosterone by mastering basics before attempting crazy hybrids seen on social media challenges. Disregarding progression risks blown ACLs from sloppy landings or Achilles tears from overzealous bounding. Build solid capacity first before chasing internet fame foolishly.

Ensure proper mobility through ankles, knees and hips critically determining capability controlling eccentric descent. If joints collapse inward or torso buckles on takeoff, regress intensity appropriately. Plyos performed correctly with sound structure remain safe for most populations.

Let's build bounce progressively, mastering bodyweight before adding load.

- **Foundational Jumps**

Start by gently prepping the nervous system and connective tissues for eventual leaping:

- **High Knees Jog**

Gradually increase pace for 30 seconds building to minutes straight. Focus on springing vertically.

- **Rocket Jumps**

Add lateral bounds side to side post high knees phase. Focus lateral push off not vertical ascent.

- **Tuck Jumps**

Raise knees to chest after competent rocket jumps phase. Avoid compromising spine arching back. Attempt single rotations initially before combos.

- **Box Jumps**

Step down, maintaining 3 points of contact. Progress height once demonstrating control.

- **Jump Squats**

Descend into a squat stance exploding upward driving arms skyward. Brace core landing softly through the hips first before knees and ankles.

Once demonstrating mastery maintaining a neutral spine during high intensity intervals above, advance into unilateral drills.

Single Leg Exercises

Splitting stance challenges smaller stabilizers improving balance and coordination simultaneously:

- Skater Hops
- Lateral Bounding
- Forward Hopping
- Backward Hopping
- Vertical Hops

Determine capacity first with bodyweight integrity before incorporating load or speed elements. This establishes proper mechanics and positions delaying fatigue bringing sloppy compensations.

Equipment Elevations

Over time begin incorporating external resistance stimulating greater ground reaction forces and metabolic demands:

Ankle Weights / Vests
Start with 1-5 lb ankle straps or lightly weighted vests to maintain proper form.

- **Plyo Boxes**

Increase box height once demonstrating controlled step downs every rep.

- **Medicine Balls**

Toss then twist catching turns simple vertical hops into whole body reactive exercises.

- **Resistance Bands**

Loop hip circles activating glutes or overhead pulls challenging upper body reactive strength.

- **Stair Running**

Skip steps integrating changed elevations. Mix sideways and backward runs too.

- **Sleds / Prowlers**

Resist driving horizontally to finish work capacity. Hand position changes hit upper or lower focus.

This gradual progression layers complexity while developing critical joint stability mobility, soft tissue compliance and skeletal density to tolerate aggressive impact long term. Be patient – years craft elite box jumpers not weeks.

In summary plyometrics fuse resistance training's strength gains with intense cardio spikes eliminating body fat in considerably shorter training duration. But respect essential progressions or face unnecessary injury risk. Hop your way to newfound confidence strutting a well earned fit and athletic physique! Just remember quality before quantity every jump session.

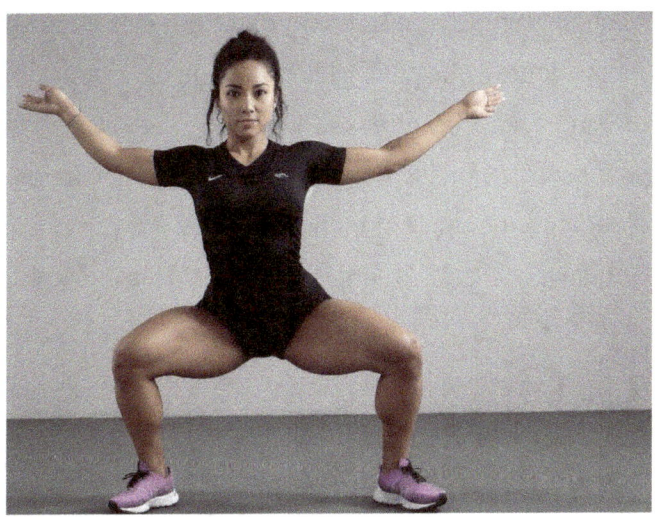

CHAPTER 9

FIND YOUR ZEN – SOOTHING YOGA FLOWS FOR RECOVERY AND MOBILITY

While prior chapters focused on intensely strengthening and shredding muscle, what goes up must come down. Building adequate rest into training balances stresses incurred breaking down tissues previously. Yoga offers ideal recovery blending gentle stretching, body awareness, breathwork and mental clarity. This chapter explores:

- Yoga benefits beyond flexibility
- Foundational pose progressions
- Beginner flow sequences

- Yoga gear useful props
- Restorative postures

Fold forward into a child's pose surrendering hectic pace giving your body TLC via calming yoga flows.

Yoga Basics

Beyond impressing (or annoying!) friends contorting into advanced pretzel poses named after dogs and birds, yoga provides numerous physical and mental health perks:

Improved flexibility

Gentle sustained stretching increases range of motion and joint mobility. Crucial for injury resilience.

Increased blood flow

Movement paired with breathing techniques enhances circulation delivering nutrients while removing waste.

Stress relief

Meditative qualities decrease nervous system hyperactivity from chronic stresses.

Mind-body awareness

Interoception and internal feedback patterns foster self study beyond the physical.

At its core hatha yoga aims harmonizing opposing energies creating balance - precisely what hard charging workout fanatics routinely lack. Let's begin laying solid foundations before attempting handstands or splits.

Foundational Poses

Ensure proper spinal alignment as priority one. While range of motion increases overtime, never sacrifice sound structure chasing depth or advanced aesthetics. Master these basic yet versatile postures first:

Downward Facing Dog

Tabletop position inverted creating spine traction and shoulder mobility. Pedal heels down stretching calves.

Pigeon Pose

Figure 4 crossing position opening hips and glutes. Use bolsters supporting the torso as needed.

Bridge Pose

Shoulder blades remain grounded lifting hips upward. Squeeze glutes at top controlling return.

Child's Pose

Relax forehead towards floor with arms extended. Opens hips and shoulders simultaneously.

Now link positions together into smooth beginner flows.

Beginner Flow Sequencing

Connecting individual poses using breath as passageway creates seamless movements orchestrating strength, flexibility and relaxation synergistically. Attempt these starter sequences:

Sun Salutations A and B

5-10 cycles moving dynamically standing to plank flows. Increases heart rate.

Neck and Shoulders
Child's pose, cat/cow, neck stretches, downward dog flows. Perfect desk job undo.

Hips Opener
Pigeon pose, figure four stretch, frog pose, bridge pose flows. Great for stiff glutes and inner thighs.

Back Relief
Kneeling cat/cow, cobra pose, locust pose, happy baby pose sequences. Soothes lumbar and thoracic tightness.

Overtime memorize transitional choreography experimenting with speed, holding stretches longer or adding repetitions building heat and intensity. Respect your limits using props like blocks or straps allowing muscles to release deeper without exceeding reasonable discomfort.

Which reminds me - support gear!

Helpful Yoga Props

Modify postures catering individual needs without forcing range lacking presently. Props like blocks, straps and bolsters serve wonderful purpose assisting proper anatomical positioning:

- Blocks - Support hips in pigeon pose or straighten arms in downward dog

- Straps - Bind around feet aiding hamstring flexibility

- Blankets - Support neck or fill gaps during seated folds

- Bolsters - Place under chest opening front body or rest torso recovering post backbends

- Chairs - Sitting option for those unable to sustain floor postures

- Sandbags - Weight atop thighs/shins during final stretches intensifying wheel or bridge poses

- Mats / Rugs - Prevent slippage and cushion joints against harder surfaces

Allowing the body fully surrendering to supportive gear creates relaxation unmatched trying to push through limitations unassisted. Now about unwinding deeper...

Restorative Postures

Concluding practice by relaxing into restorative elements permits healing benefits saturating mind, body and spirit wholly. Extended holds using numerous props blends gentle stretching with meditation:

Legs Up Wall Pose

Inverts against the wall benefiting low back similar to forward folds but less intense.

Supported Fish Pose

Bolsters stacked enable spine extending without strain.

Blanket Nested Child's Pose
Sensory experience comforting as a baby cradled tightly.

Yin Seated Forward Bend
Softens hamstrings, lower back and releases neck tension.

Savasana Corpse Pose
Close eyes fully melting into the support surface without effort.

By consciously slowing pace and eliminating effort, true realization washes over how little required attaining happiness and inner peace. Yoga cleanses internal clutter welcoming present moment awareness. Keep breaths steady allowing your next exhale fully cleansing stresses away. practice letting go. Welcome lighter embodiment.

CHAPTER 10

EXTREME CONDITIONING - HIIT AND TABATA BLASTERS

Looking to send fat cells scattering while transforming workout productivity tenfold? Then it's time to embrace the dark arts of metabolic conditioning! Extreme exercise protocols like high intensity interval training (HIIT) and Tabata workouts leverage science behind superior conditioning driving unprecedented changes upgrading bodies rapidly.

We overview:
- HIIT background
- Equipment options

- Tabata formatting
- Hybrid strength combos
- Additional protocols

Strap in and secure all belongings during this turbulent chapter guaranteed to shake fitness complacency launching results into hyperdrive!

HIIT Explained

Steady paced medium intensity cardio definitely burns calories during exercise but fails igniting maximal post exercise oxygen consumption (EPOC) underutilizing slower fat burning mechanisms after training ceases. High intensity interval training fixes this flaw.

Think repeated bouts of maximum intensity effort followed by short rest before the next all-out work stage again. By spiking exertion beyond lactate threshold quickly, oxygen debt rapidly accumulates. What follows may resemble temporary death but metabolic disturbance remains. The aftermath incinerates calories for hours as the body restores homeostasis. Talk about afterburn!

But isn't this risky? Won't overdoing interval intensity increase injury or burnout? Certainly overzealous application harms but strategically prescribed the benefits outweigh hypotheticals. Let exercise science soothe fears.

Evidence confirms HIIT enhances mitochondrial density and cardiovascular function beyond moderate intensity training while requiring considerably less weekly duration. Vastly improved conditioning and body composition changes occur working smarter not harder. But first master move mechanics and control avoiding sloppy form fatigue brings later on. Let's overview proper equipment preparations next.

Equipment Options

Traditional cardio machines definitely suffice creating intervals. But why limit explosive efforts battling inertia from wheels or belts? Use equipment allowing unrestricted maximal speed and mobility. Consider:

Bodyweight circuits

Burpees, jump squats, mountain climbers, suicide sprints - athletic drills translate well opening unlimited creativity designing evil complexes.

Kettlebells

Ballistics like swings, cleans and snatches blend strength and power simultaneously.

Medicine balls

Slams, chop rotations and throws across open spaces crank intensity.

Resistance bands

Anchor above head for battling pull downs or around knees during lateral walks.

Prowler sleds

Resisted sprinting presses metabolic limits quickly. Vary direction and hand positions.

Jacobs ladders

Climbing vertical treadmills spikes heart rates exponentially.

Each option allows seamless transition from max efforts to reduced active rest periods. Now let's examine structured interval protocols more closely.

Tabata Intervals

Developed by Japanese scientist Dr. Izumi Tabata, this ruthless template pushes four minute suffering thresholds maximizing conditioning gains documented in research studies. Simply:

20 seconds maximum intensity
10 seconds complete rest
Repeat 8 cycles total (4 minutes)

Traditionally bodyweight exercises like burpees or kettlebell swings worked best but as fitness industry evolved so have applications:

Strength Tabatas:
Heavy thrusters, dumbbell snatches, compound lifts

Machine Tabatas:
Rowers, versa climbers, airdyne bikes

Calisthenics Tabatas:

Mountain climbers, jump squats, high knees

The short duration facilitates going full throttle each round knowing rest arrives shortly. This permits maintaining peak exertion consistently versus pacing over longer durations. Completing multiple Tabatas with different movements torches calories for monster EPOC payoffs melting fat for hours afterwards.

Term confusion exists between HIIT and Tabata but simply put:

HIIT = Interval intensity over longer periods
Tabata = Structured 20/10 format for 4 minutes

Now enhance potency blending moves together.

Mashed Up Hybrids

Combine strength lifts with intense cardio accelerating conditioning gains evolving classic protocols:

- Complexes: Cycle 6-8 moves fluidly with zero rest until all complete. Repeat 3-5x.

- Density Training: Specify time cap i.e. 6 minutes maxing reps of 1-2 moves. Record RPE (rate of perceived exertion) and heart rate trends.

- AMRAP: As many rounds/reps as possible in a given time frame - great for pairing ladder routines or descending pyramid schemes.

- Chipper Workouts: Series of exercises ending with miserable high rep isolation like 100 squats or mountain climbers. Sadistic!

Many apps create customizable WODs (workouts of the day) automatically programming varied movements, rest intervals and rounds. This adds novelty keeping motivation high. Speaking of apps...

Apps / Timers

Monitoring interval precision guarantees optimal quality and consistent improvement versus sloppy execution or primitive estimations. Apps like:

- Gymboss - programs customizable rounds and rest periods

- Seconds Pro - create multiple clocks with labels

- JEFIT - huge database for recording workouts

- Tabata Songs - music timed perfectly

Most exercise equipment and watches contain internal timers also useful should technology fail you. Back to the old faithful stopwatch works fine too!

With arsenal fully stocked adding extreme training diversity let's finish surveying additional methods for future experimentation.

Bonus Interval Protocols

Beyond Tabata and classic HIIT, plenty of additional formats offer slight variations. Among the more popular:

EMOM

Every minute on the minute perform a set task working for the rest of 60 seconds. Allows managing fatigue.

Heart Rate Intervals

Use percentage max heart rate determining work/rest periods. Spares guesswork.

Navy Seal Training

4-5 cycles 300 yard sprints, 100 push ups, 100 sit ups, 20 pull ups. Sadistic!

Fartlek Training

Swedish term meaning "speedplay". Random intervals based on feel and terrain. Used often by runners.

Many options exist bending classic interval training around life's realities and limitations. Remain diligent tracking stress effects avoiding burnout. Cycle intensity allows proper recovery to recharge for subsequent weeks. Find optimal sustainable frequency through trial and error. Program small training blocks dedicated attacking weaknesses obstructing goals. But remain patient - Rome wasn't built in a day and neither will be your ultimate physique or fitness level. Trust the consistency compounds progress exponentially over enough time.

The formula works when applied prudently. So let's collectively step up taking on the challenge of improving daily 1% at a time. Progress awaits!

CHAPTER 11

REBUILD AND RECOVER - ESSENTIAL RESTORATION FOR PROGRESS

Following intense training bouts breaking down muscle, organized recovery protocols help facilitate adaptation critical for ongoing gains. Skipping cool-downs or neglecting self-care sabotages progress made by busting butt previously. Consistent training demands calculated easing off periods we will overview:

- Cool-down basics
- Foam rolling benefits
- Stretching science
- Restorative yoga
- Lifestyle factors
- Additional modalities

Let's skillfully balance taxing and relaxing allowing fitter, faster versions emerging long-term.

Why Cooling Down Matters

Gradually easing exertion levels at the end of exercise provides multiple benefits:

- Lessens delayed onset muscle soreness (DOMS)
- Returns heart rate baseline preventing dizziness
- Removes metabolic waste products pooling in tissue
- Transitions nervous system fire back to parasympathetic rest
- Mentally closes effort and begins recovery

Think of it as slowly easing off the gas after flooring your sports car around the track. You wouldn't recklessly brake suddenly – treat your body with similar care. Building this ritual solidifies gains made each training while optimizing restoration.

Cool-Down Essentials

Dedicate 5-10 minutes at the conclusion of every training session transitioning exertion back towards normalcy. Methods include:

Light Cardio

Walk laps or pedal easily allowing heart rate and breathing slowing. Signals workout complete.

Foam Rolling

Applying pressure loosening tight areas pools waste and signals blood flow to neglected zones.

Static Stretching

Gentle lengthening of actively worked prime movers increases pliability.

Breathwork

Box breathing or alternate nostril breathing rebalances the nervous system shifting back to rest.

The combination circulates nutrient rich blood, removes inflammatory acids and relaxes structures for tissue remodeling later on. Now let's break down the self-myofascial release next.

Benefits of Foam Rolling

That pleasurable yet awkward act of applying body weight pressure kneading tight spots helps muscles and fascia release stored tension. Using tools like foam rollers or lacrosse balls creates localized compression forcing tense areas to expand. Benefits include:

- Break up trigger points
- Improve range of motion
- Removes lactic acid buildup
- Increases blood flood
- Reduces muscle soreness
- Frees bound nerves

Roll gently 90 seconds per zone before or after training – inner thighs, calves, lats, chest, low back, glutes. Let discomfort guide pressure levels targeting denser gathering spots. Breathe slowly as tissues begin surrendering tightness.

Now about stretching...

Stretching Strategies

While foam rolling targets myofascial layers surrounding muscles, static stretching aims to lengthen muscle tissue itself. Gentle sustained pulling increases flexibility and mobility:

- Reduces stiffness and soreness
- Improves coordination
- Prevents overuse injuries
- Realigns posture
- Releases bound nerves
- Enhances mind-body connection

Focus large muscle groups at the conclusion of sessions – hips, hamstrings, chest, shoulders. Use straps if lacking range of motion reaching toes or hands together. Prioritizing function over IG likes attempting advanced poses.

30-60 seconds per muscle 2-3 repetitions expands range of motion noticeably over weeks. For whole body restorative stretching try beginner friendly yoga flows.

Restorative Yoga Flows

Linking gentle poses together into a moving meditation provides passive stretching holding deeper stretches conveniently. Sequences may include:

- Child's pose to cat/cow to downward dog
- Forward fold to standing side bend
- Low lunge to half pigeon
- Bridge to supine twist

Emphasis lies grounding fully into each posture using gravity optimally rather than force. Breathe slowly into tight areas without exceeding reasonable discomfort. Use props like bolsters to support the body allowing surrender.

These tranquil flows reduce resting muscle tension and heart rates while stimulating parasympathetic relaxation. When combined with proper lifestyle factors outside the gym, transformative regeneration occurs.

Lifestyle Recovery Factors

Supplementing mechanical interventions optimizing recovery involves dialing in daily habits complementing fitness efforts:

- Hydration - Halve body weight(lbs) Drink minimum fluid ounces daily from water and herbal teas

- Nutrition - Emphasize anti-inflammatory whole foods - fatty fish, vegetables, healthy fats from avocados, nuts and seeds. Limit inflammatory refined grains, sugars and alcohol.

- Sleep - Average 7-9 hours nightly. Keep consistent times. Limit blue light and digital stimulation after 8pm.

- Stress modulation - Try meditation, laughter yoga, forest bathing or float tanks quieting chronic stressors hampering gains.

These simple suggestions reduce drag on the body from less than ideal lifestyle inputs. But we can target recovery even greater with additional holistic modalities like:

Supplemental Modalities

Experiment incorporating extra elements fine tuning restoration for amplified adaptation between sessions:

- Cryotherapy chambers
- Flotation therapy
- Dry needling/cupping
- Sports massages
- Chiropractic adjustments
- Infrared saunas

Each assumes supporting roles repairing injury sites, reducing soreness or speeding waste removal complementary traditional training itself.

Be proactive programming ample TLC for your body beyond brutal workouts themselves. Consider cooling down rituals and lifestyle optimization setting the table for muscle magic manifesting during rest afterwards. Healing happens during downtime between sessions - make the most by optimizing rejuvenation with these proven tips!

Consistency remains king but recovery proves queen empowering long term gains. All hail the queen!

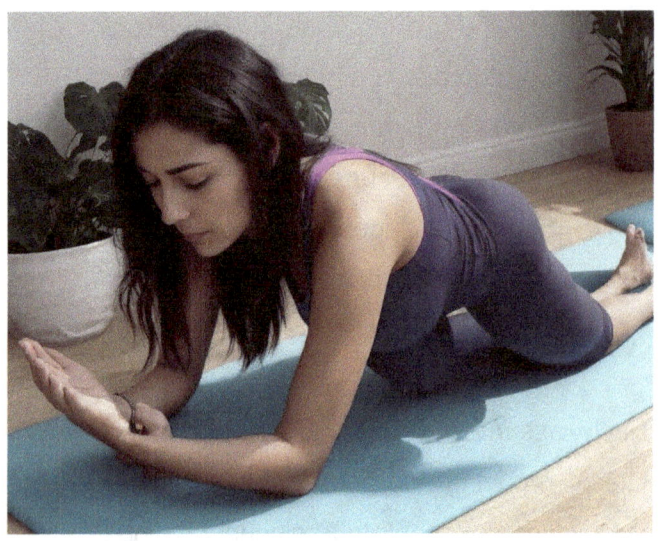

CHAPTER 12

FUEL FOR FAT LOSS - CRAFTING A BODY TRANSFORMATION DIET

Exercise serves as the stimulus but food fuels the physique. Without proper nutritional inputs supporting training, aesthetic goals stall short despite Herculean efforts previously. But fear not - small meal planning tweaks generate BIG aesthetic and performance benefits!

I'll overview:

- Caloric basics
- Macronutrient targets
- Meal timing strategies
- Sample meal plans
- Crucial considerations
- Bonus fat loss tips

Let's start cooking noticeable improvements maximizing your genetic potential!

Caloric Basics

Before modifying food quality, sufficient quantity forms the nutritional foundation. While old school "eat less, exercise more" gets parroted endlessly, best practices prioritize retaining metabolism-stoking muscle mass while shredding fat stores specifically.

Calculate a baseline caloric need starting point using the Mifflin St Jeor equation factoring current weight, height, age and gender. For females:

$$BMR = (9.99 \times \text{weight in kg}) + (6.25 \times \text{height in cm}) - (4.92 \times \text{age}) - 161$$

This approximates necessary calories for basal functioning ignoring activity levels. Increase daily calories from 15-30% based on your training frequency and intensity. For example:

Sedentary office worker = BMR x 1.15
Moderate exerciser (3 days/week) = BMR x 1.25
Athlete (6+ intense sessions/week) = BMR x 1.3

Track averages over weeks ensuring weight trends downwards between 0.5-1% of total mass weekly maximum. Losing 1-2 lbs weekly nets better long term results than extreme deficits losing 6-8 lbs monthly which risks metabolic damage.

Trust the process of adjusting intake based on body feedback and performance in the gym, not rigid theory. Sample ranges simply guide initial targets.

Macronutrient Manipulation
Next optimize food quality balancing proper protein muscle growth, fats to steady hormone production and carbs to fuel intense training demands. General starting ranges include:

Protein – 1.6-2.2 g per kg bodyweight
Fats – 30% total calories
Carbohydrates – Remainder of calories

We will customize these further but for now simply monitor hitting minimums, especially protein while remaining in caloric deficit range determined previously. High protein diets aid fat loss efforts in numerous research studies compared to traditional low fat/high carb approaches. Time to sample plans!

Sample Meal Plan

Here is what properly balanced targeted fat loss nutrition may entail for a 150 lb female training 4 days per week:

Daily Calories: 1900

Protein Minimum: 120 g (480 calories)

Fat Minimum: 70 g (630 calories)

Remaining Carbs/Protein: 190 g (760 calories)

Breakfast

3 eggs, 2 cups spinach, 1/2 avocado

Lunch

8 oz chicken, 1 cup rice, 1 cup vegetables

Dinner

8 oz salmon, Sweet potato, Asparagus

Snacks

Greek yogurt, Mixed berries, Pistachios

This simplified template hits proper ratios starting around 30% protein, 30% fat, 40% carbs microscopically. Tweak to individual taste but ensure protein minimums to maintain muscle mass through the fat loss phase.

Now personalize further dialing nutrition strategically.

Custom Considerations

While the basics serve most populations well starting out, nuance nutrition based on:

- Training demands
- Digestive tolerances
- Lifestyle factors
- Economic limitations

For example:

1) Cyclists require greater carbs than powerlifters

2) Those sensitive digesting beans or dairy steer towards alternative protein sources

3) Busy professionals value convenient meal prep over elaborate cooking

4) Budget conscious shoppers plan cost efficient nutrition tactics

Again embrace flexibility finding YOUR customized fat loss formula through journaling and gauging progress weekly. Now for icing on the cake, accelerating results...

Accelerated Fat Loss Tips

No fitness guide would be complete without including common effective strategies speeding fat disappearance leveraging science:

- Caffeine - Enjoy black coffee pre-training maximizing fat utilization during sessions

- Green Tea - Powerful antioxidant optimizing health and slight metabolism boost

- Resistance Training - Weights/circuits build calorie burning muscle improving body composition

- NEAT training - Take walks after meals, fidget during workdays, take stairs whenever possible

- Intermittent Fasting - Restrict eating window to 8 hours daily improving insulin sensitivity

- High Protein - Retain/build muscle so increasing dietary protein proves key

- Water Intake - Hydration optimizes bodily functions aiding fat metabolism and reducing false hunger signals

The root fundamentals craft body transformations, but these additions provide nice complementary perks. Just don't complicate it before mastering the basics first.

In summary balanced nutrition supporting fuel needs particularly protein provisions retains hard earned muscle mass while moderate caloric deficits drains unwanted fat stores specifically. Trust the calculators initially before custom tailoring to individual preference maximizing adherence and progress towards dream physiques!

CHAPTER 13

BEYOND THE BASICS - 12 WEEK STRENGTH PROGRAM

Congratulations attempting more advanced programming graduating beyond initial beginner work! Consistently applying sound bodyweight principles crafts increasingly more capable bodies. Now further those fitness foundations with a formal 12 week strength cycle intentionally progressing quantitative workload sensitively without overdoing too quickly.

This chapter provides:

- Training split rationale
- Exercise menu ideas
- Detailed schedule
- Progression tactics
- Deload necessity
- Sample exercises

Let's strategically sculpt our strongest physique ever!

Training Split Explanation

Rather than hastily attacking the gym haphazardly each visit, an organized training split based on movement patterns and muscle group pairings optimizes results by:

- Allowing proper recovery between sessions
- Preventing overuse injuries from redundancy
- Maximizing effort and focus each session

Our split example will use:

Lower body
Core + cardio conditioning
Upper horizontal push
Upper horizontal pull
Upper vertical push
Upper vertical pull
Rest

This balances anatomy emphasizing opposing muscle groups each session to meet strength goals quicker. Let's map out the details.

12 Week Overview

Our phase entails 3 mesocycles each lasting 4 microcycles. Each microcycle iterates adding load or volume. By month's end recovery allows supercompensation preparing subsequent progressive waves:

Phase 1 (Weeks 1-4)

Establish baseline strength. Focus perfect form through higher reps before increasing load.

Phase 2 (Weeks 4-8)

Increase intensity early each microcycle either adding weight, speed or reduced rest breaks.

Phase 3 (Weeks 9-12)

Maximize strength pushing limits before reduced load deload week.

Each period stresses the body uniquely to spur adaptation best responded with strategic recovery. Let's examine individual sessions.

Daily Workouts

Lower Body Strength
Focus barbell squats, trap bar deadlifts, split squats, hip thrusts, challenging legs and glutes.

Core + Conditioning
Alternate heavy farmers walks with core barbell movements. Finish intervals targeting weaknesses.

Horizontal Push
Barbell bench variations, weighted dips, fly movements.

Horizontal Pull
Barbell rows, chest supported rows, and pull .

Vertical Push
Shoulder barbell presses, handstand push-ups, Arnold presses.

Vertical Pull

Pull ups, inverted rows, face pulls emphasizing upper back.

Rest Day

Active recovery only - light cardio, stretching, foam rolling.

This balanced plan progresses by overloading each microcycle without allowing CNS excess fatigue through built-in off days. Now increase difficulty sensibly.

Progression Tactics

Improving any physical quality requires gradually progressing stimulus levels as capacity increases. Carefully channel added workload minimizing injury risk:

Weight / Load

Increase conservatively first ensuring movement patterns are mastered without compensation. Start loads very light!

Repetitions

Add reps before bumping the load significantly. Ensure completing final sets near muscular failure with sound form.

Speed / Tempo

Once comfortable with strict reps, quicken pace with consistency is still a priority. Explosive days balance controlled days.

Rest Periods

Trim rest intervals between sets to increase density and time tension on target areas. Monitor technique closely as fatigue mounts.

Range of Motion

Gradually descend deeper into squats or pull higher on vertical presses mobilizing joints safely.

With patience, stress and recovery balance even among advanced athletes. Periodization allows adaptation and renewed progress consistently compared to chaotic undisciplined programs attempted frequently.

Deloading Necessity

After several weeks of progressive loading, a deload week halving intensity proves wise recharging the nervous system and nagging joint pains often accumulating. Here is simplified deloading template:

- All exercises - Half intensity, stop sets prior failure by a few reps, reduce load, sets and volume significantly.

- Emphasis - Move slowly with mindfulness maintaining perfect technical execution every rep.

- Sessions - Keep total under one hour with minimal conditioning elements included.

The idea lies in allowing tissues and the central nervous system fully recovering before the next demanding meso begins. Light technique rehearsal refines motor patterns also. Now sample what exercises may populate sessions.

Sample Exercise Selection

While entire programming exceeds our chapter scope, the below menu serves filling each session effectively. Modify or substitute alternatives catering specific needs or limitations present:

Lower Power

Back squats, trap bar deadlifts, hip thrusters, sled sprints

Core + Conditioning

Hanging leg raise, ab wheel rollout, sled push, battling ropes

Horizontal Push

Barbell bench press, weighted push ups, dumbbell flyes

Horizontal Pull

Bent over rows, chest supported rows, inverted rows

Vertical Push

Overhead barbell press, Arnold press, handstand push ups

Vertical Pull

Pull ups, lat pulldowns, inverted rows, face pulls

Cardio / Vanity

Elliptical intervals, heavy bag, muscle rounds

Using the above framework as template, this phase stratifies proper workload maximizing strength expressible through purposeful undulating stress. By adjusting volume, intensity and exercise selection each phase, progressive overload sustains lifting heavier weights and technical prowess long term. What separates average and elite performers? Consistency and the ability to limit failure. Plan ahead scheduling success.

In closing, I pursue monthly metrics checking my ego. Accumulate tension judiciously to avoid tipping too far, braking systems down completely. Balance training dosage alongside life's demands outside the gym proactively. The secret of making lasting gains inevitable? Simply showing up...1% better daily. Now let's get growing!

CHAPTER 14

STAYING POWER – SUSTAINING CONSISTENCY AND MOTIVATION

The fitness journey entails endless micro decisions either inching closer toward goals or rationalizing backward steps. While inspiration fuels initial enthusiasm, maintaining Determination separates dabblers from champions. This chapter provides tactics strengthening resilience powering through motivational ruts and plateaus inevitably arising.

We will cover:
- Goal setting psychology
- Plateaus troubleshooting
- Scheduling workarounds
- Tracking progress
- Support communities
- Rewarding milestones

Let's sustain consistency upgrading fitness lifestyles permanently, not just yearly January 1st rebounds!

Goal Setting Strategies

Vague aspirations like "get in shape" lack the detail driving lasting change. Transform nebulous dreams into S.M.A.R.T goals:

- Specific - Quantify the who, what, when, where, why portions precisely.

- Measurable – Include numeric amounts gauging achievement definitively.

- Attainable – Challenge slightly beyond current ability promoting growth.

- Relevant – Ensure your "why" emotionally connects goals to core values.

- Time-bound – Specify deadlines creating urgency and benchmarks.

Well defined S.M.A.R.T goals provide clarity missing meandering aimlessly through workouts lacking purpose. Review and revise regularly. Now about overcoming plateaus...

Plateaus and Rebounds

After initial novice gains are earned quickly, progression stagnates suddenly despite concerted efforts. More advanced levels require finely tuned details lifting performance. Break plateaus incorporating:

- Deload weeks – Reduce volume allowing the body to fully recover. Reboot fresh.

- Periodization – Vary training variables using organized load, volume and intensity fluctuations.

- Weakness targeting – Isolate lagging muscle groups with focused sessions.

- Nutrition adjustments – Review dietary adherence and recovery practices hampering progress.

- Patience, perseverance – Trust delayed transformation still unfolds through consistency.

Plateaus generate frustration but indicate readiness advancing beyond current thresholds. Embrace redesign necessities and upgrade programming thoughtfully.

Now build margin balancing life's unpredictability.

Schedule With Flexibility

Rigid regimens quickly unravel confronting inevitable life obligations. Allow flexibility cushioning workouts week to week:

- Off Day Floaters – Float 1-2 off days weekly adjusting to unexpected events.

Split Sessions – Break workouts across morning and evening if time crunched.

- Home Backups – Keep resistance bands, kettlebells, suspended trainers for remote training needs.

- Calendar Reviews – Touchbase start each week optimizing forthcoming days proactively.

- Unfinished Effort – Complete unfinished workouts before starting new ones if interrupted suddenly.

Preserve training infrastructure first before worrying isolation exercise omissions. Perfect never should impede good enough. Now track progress not just problems!

Progress Tracking

What improves measured improves management. Monitoring key indicators informs needed adjustments optimizing future sessions:

- Workout Logging – Document exercises, sets, reps, load and weekly volume trends.

- Body Metrics – Track weight, body fat percentage, circumferences revealing physique changes.

- Mobility Markers – Record range of motion, movement competency improvements.

- Performance PRs – Celebrate personal records like 5k times or 1 rep maxes.

- Photo Comparisons – Visually inspect monthly physique changes side by side.

Data guides more than motivates. But surrounding oneself by like minded supportive communities generates momentum also.

Encouraging Communities
Isolating while pursuing intimidating fitness goals feels draining quick. Connect frequently with

positive social groups reinforcing identity and growth:

- Gym Friends – Bond pushing each other during early morning or evening regulars.

- Family Allies – Enlist personal cheerleaders believing your vision helps navigate life's hiccups.

Online Forums – Reddit, Facebook and niche blogs offer digital comrades pursuing similar dreams.

- Coaches / Mentors – Invest in experienced coaches customizing guidance through personalized services or premade programs.

Everyone needs that occasional pull, spotting danger, or reality check reaching aspirations independently unsuccessfully otherwise. Now accelerate efforts rewarding little wins consistently.

Milestone Rewards

Reinforce small behaviors keeping momentum steering progress in the right direction via planned rewards:

- Massages – Schedule restorative bodywork realigning tissues and energy leveling up recovery.

- Nutritious Meals – Savor wholesome nutrient dense meals refueling properly without guilt sabotaging progress.

- Inspiring Events – Attend workshops, seminars or conferences with world class experts elevating games.

- Explorative Adventures – Embark bucket list activities as checkpoints celebrating consistency paying off.

- Gear Upgrades – Upgrade shoes, heart rate monitors, workout apparel that functionally serve beyond simply looking cool.

Attach incentives recognizing consistency gaining traction. But avoid unhealthy temptations undoing progress. The process remains the prize, not just goal achievement.

In closing fitness level caps our human potential and life's experience directly hinging health. Commit to lifelong betterment for not only looking better temporarily but functioning optimally daily. What vehicles transport you confidently through the next seasons of life ahead? Inspiration moves the body but consistency transforms the body.

CHAPTER 15

TRAINING THROUGH INJURY - SMART EXERCISE MODIFICATIONS FOR OPTIMAL RECOVERY

Inevitably in any fitness journey, injury or joint pain can emerge disrupting training consistency. Whether from overuse, poor mechanics or freak accidents, working around physical limitations protects hard-earned progress rather than losing ground recovering. This chapter explores smart training adjustments, gentle rehab and seeking professional help strategically.

We'll cover:
- Respecting pain signals
- Modifying workouts safely
- Rehabilitation exercises
- Seeking health experts
- Nutritional support
- Stress reduction

By responding judiciously, comebacks manifest stronger having endured this storm before. Let's rebuild sensibly earning capability and resilience facing future setbacks with confidence.

Respecting Pain Signals

Attempting to mask discomfort with stubborn grit while continuing training often backfires, exacerbating damage and delaying proper healing. Instead develop bodily awareness identifying dysfunction early:

- Evaluate movement patterns during warm-ups for compensation changes suggesting imbalances or instability.
- Note pain levels during workouts using a 1-10 scale, modifying or stopping completely exceeding 3-4.
- Recognize pain onset timing - immediate or accumulating gradually over time.

Let symptoms guide training adjustments respectfully. Next modify activities staying active as able based on realistic pain-free capabilities.

Smart Training Modifications

Rather than complete rest, adjust variables per tolerance while maintaining consistency benefiting recovery:

- Lower intensity lessening weight, sets and reps based on movement capability pain-free
- Lengthen repetition duration emphasizing slow negatives less taxing than explosive positives
- Widen rest intervals allowing greater muscle recovery between sets
- Reduce range of motion higher or lower minimizing joint angles provoking pain
- Eliminate specific aggravating exercises completely if all above fail alleviating symptoms

Preserving training habits supports patients psychologically while preventing muscle loss or conditioning erosion typical when abstaining completely. But strategic rehab exercises also restore function quicker.

Rehabilitation Exercises

Address problematic areas with targeted corrective work like:

- Foam rolling knots releasing muscles bound down hypertonically
- Stretching tight, overactive muscles reestablishing reciprocal inhibition balance
- Activating weak, inhibited muscles gradually rebuilding joint integrity
- Massaging trigger points or cross-frictioning scar tissue adhesions
- Attempting gentle progressive range of motion movements loading affected areas without sharp pains

The adage "motion is lotion" proves effective restoring mobility to injured joints, tendons and surrounding tissues. Respect symptoms by dialing intensity aligning capability, not ego.

Now identify when professional help warrants consideration.

Seeking Health Experts

While self-management suffices minor tweaks, serious trauma like torn muscles or broken bones requires prompt medical intervention. Seek help if experiencing:

- Extreme swelling/bruising
- Visibly deformed joints/limbs
- Inability weight bearing through affected area
- Locked/fixed joints lacking normal mobility
- Loss of muscle strength or sensations like tingling/numbness

Consulting physical therapists, sports medicine doctors or orthopedists proves wise navigating diagnosis details and guided recovery plans. Therapeutic modalities like laser, graston, e-stim or dry needling effectively address trickier issues like scar tissue or chronic inflammation.

An ounce of prevention overrides pounds of cure however. Support full recovery further through nutrition.

Nutritional Support

Diet optimizing protein intake, micronutrient density and anti-inflammatory balance helps injured bodies mend quicker:

- Protein - Increase intake up to 2 grams per kilogram body weight supplying amino acid building blocks remodeling damaged tissues.
- Micronutrients - Vital minerals like magnesium, zinc and B vitamins aid cellular repair communicating proper chemical signals optimizing function.
- Anti-inflammatories - Reduce inflammatory fats, sugars and grains. Increase natural compounds like turmeric, omega 3s and vitamin C.
- Hydration - Thirst cues underestimate fluid losses. Measure water intake targeting half

bodyweight (lbs) in minimum daily fluid ounces.

Fine tuning nutrition removes roadblocks stalling otherwise seamless comebacks. But overcoming emotional barriers proves equally effective.

Stress and Mindset Care

Injuries shake identity and derail best laid plans overwhelming even disciplined athletes. Seek support reestablishing empowering perspective during low moments:

- Connect frequently with positive social groups reinforcing self-concept regardless physical state
- Journal progress celebrating subtle daily wins however minor recognizing healing manifested
- Consider setbacks temporary opportunities redirecting training, nutrition and recovery practices for the better long-term

- Appreciate enforced breaks from extreme chronic training levels previously as reset allowing greater capacity later
- Embrace limitations self-compassionately without judgment knowing comebacks await on the other side

An optimistic yet realistic mindset endures storms regaining momentum faster. Have hope and faith - this too shall pass.

In conclusion consistently applying adjustments above minimizes lost progress or psychological despair. Reclaim health maximizing all resources expediting daily recovery. Dedicate restoring complete function before chasing former bests or comparison with others. Patience through this process returns better than before if trust and self-compassion persists. We endured storms before, we will again. You've got this!

CONCLUSION

Reclaiming Your Strongest, Leanest Body Yet

After exploring beginner concepts plus advanced training philosophies through this journey together, your reinforced foundational fitness knowledge positions progress unobstructed moving forward. Commend yourself for prioritizing personal health despite busyness tempting conveniently otherwise. Remember the fastest results craft not from extreme effort bursts but sustainable systems compounding gains consistently in the long run.

This manual aimed condensing mixed fitness information into digestible fitness fundamentals benefiting women specifically. Through sample workouts, targeted nutritional guidance and lifestyle design upgrades, transpose book inspiration into daily personal practices. What sticks determines destiny more than what is temporarily stimulating.

Trust the process. Have patience with your body and believe in your inner abilities transforming. Because small hinges swing big doors and tiny gains accumulate into massive personal revolutions in due time. Keep watering the seeds planted through this program until blooming inevitably.

Now pull everything together into actionable steps enriching your life's seasons positively regardless of age or limitations faced previously.

Call to Action

If beginning fitness awakening feels intimidating alone initially, lean on book guidance getting started correctly. Lifelong health spans beyond single program experience. Allow this catalyst sparking fitter existence through:

Realistic Goal Setting

Inchstones build empires. Set modest realistic metrics steering accomplishments ahead.

Smaller Habits

Attempt manageable consistent actions summing giant results.

Accountability

Surround yourself by supportive communities fostering growth.

Tenacity

When lacking motivation, discipline bridges gaps inconsistently otherwise.

Self Compassion

Progress not perfection keeps perspective realistic amid setbacks.

You stand capable now lifting body optimism further. But should questions or uncertainty resurface later, reference book materials solidifying knowledge into habitual practice. Also reach out and share your journey with others.

Now available - Paperback copies for easier bookmarked reference revisiting workout templates, nutritional recommendations and lifestyle upgrades most relevant confiscating excuses previously rationalized.

Secure your physical copy today through Amazon print copy services:

Lastly before parting, if you found this program effective please also rate the book positively on Amazon encouraging other women benefiting similarly building happier fitness habits. Progress multiplies passing wisdom onto others and pays it forward!

Now confidently walk forward constantly bettering daily. Because small hinges swing big doors and tiny gains accumulate into massive personal revolutions in due time. You stand more prepared, strengthening your body and life's trajectory positively through fitness world truths. Be proud of the commitment toward self improvement prioritizing greater personal capability and healthier living ahead. Keep seeking growth through patience and trust. Believe in your abilities transforming - the best remains out there still.

Onward and upward always!

AUTHOR NOTE

Congratulations reaching the final page of our empowering fitness journey together! As a bestselling fitness author and magazine contributor, I aim to create digestible training and nutrition guides benefiting time-strapped women specifically.

This manual condensed proven strategies upgrading readers' trajectories positively. Through sample workouts, targeted nutritional recommendations and lifestyle design best practices, I hope you feel equipped to progress in self-improvement further. What wisdom resonates most confiscating excuses previously rationalized? Apply those elements first before worrying about incorporating each detail simultaneously. Tiny gains accumulate into massive revolutions extended over time if we persistently sow seeds through perpetual daily 1% betterment.

I wrote this book wishing I had access to simplified training approaches maximizing limited gym durations when first overhauling my own mediocre physique and health years ago as an overworked fitness professional initially. May this manual accelerate your success avoiding unnecessary trial-and-error while maximizing genetics fully.

Now available - Paperback copies for easier bookmarked reference revisiting workout templates, nutritional recommendations and lifestyle upgrades whenever motivation dips or uncertainty resurfaces later down road. Secure your physical copy today through Amazon print copy services allowing notes scribbled further customizing approach most relevant overcoming personal limitations:

How can you help this body transformation guide reach other aspiring women similarly? Please rate the book positively on Amazon encouraging future improved editions refined by your much appreciated feedback. Progress multiplies passing wisdom onto others paying goodness forward!

In closing, allow me to thank you personally for investing time and financial resources into your betterment and this created work. May elevated energy levels, positlve physique enhancements and lifestyle design upgrades manifest abundantly sowing efforts here towards external impact there. Please reach out and share your journey with myself and others. Together we lift as iron sharpens iron towards individual and shared greatness collectively. I cheer you onward wholeheartedly!

Now confidently walk forward constantly bettering daily. You stand more prepared, strengthening your body and life's trajectory by positively applying truths within. Be proud of prioritizing greater health and capability ahead. Greater awaits those persevering patiently through small progress compounded over time. Keep seeking growth through trust; believe in your inner abilities transforming - the best remains out there still. Onward and upward always!

[RICHARD L. LYONS]

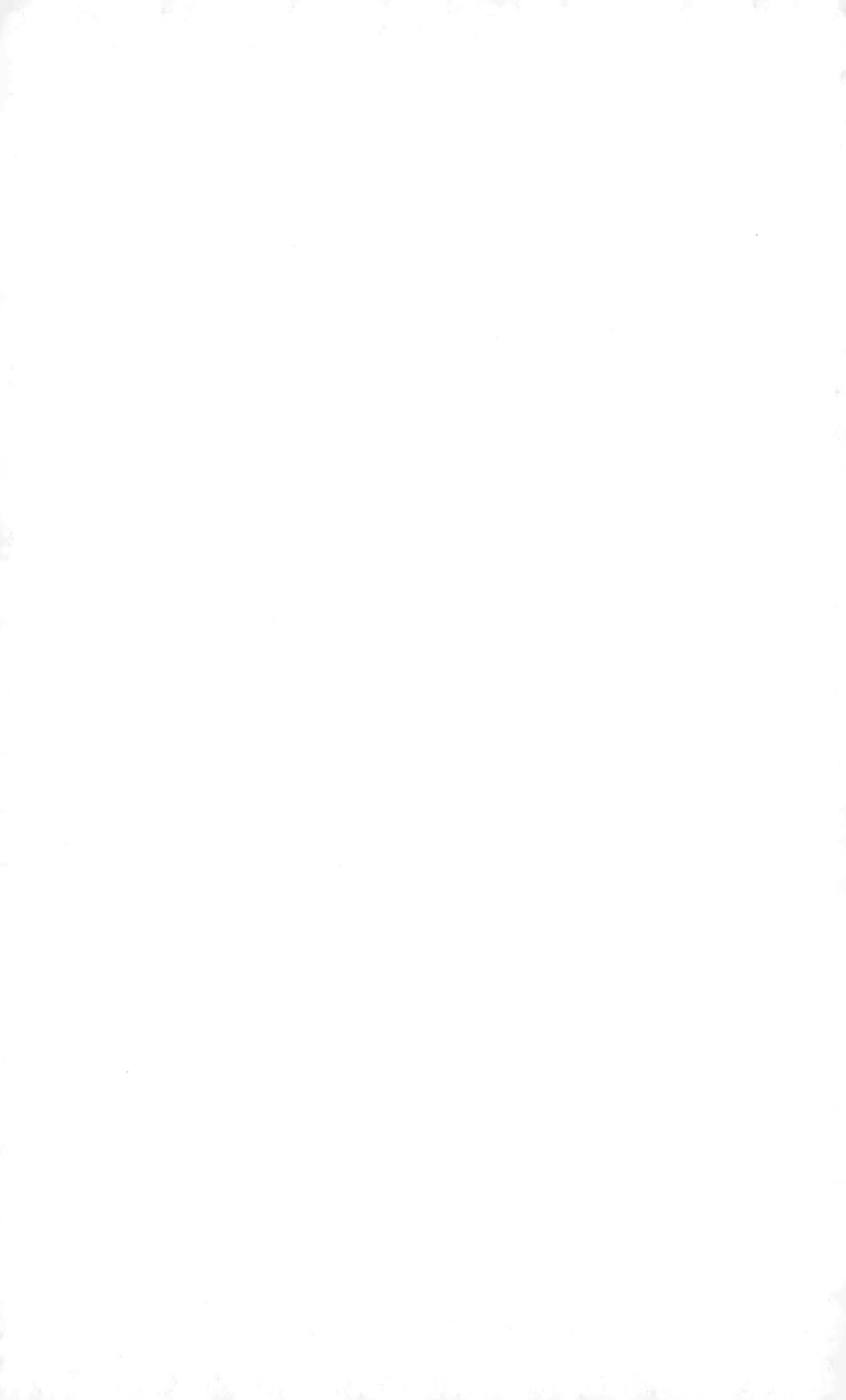